It's Your Health –

OWN IT

Diary of a Family and Food Allergies

Vandester J Jenkins

ISBN-10: 1512354856
ISBN-13: 978-1512354850

DEDICATION

To my parents, Constance and Hugh, who have always supported my dreams and encouraged my pursuits. And to all the parents out there who know what it's like to worry from, dawn to dusk, about the health and well-being of their children, yet willingly go the extra mile to see that their little ones live, thrive, and be happy.

WHY THIS BOOK

The entire reason for this book is to get the discussions going on allergies and the impact to a person's health. I claim no professional knowledge of allergies and how to treat them, only my personal experiences on how I have dealt with them. And in this book, I wanted you to be able to compare how they may or may not be similar to your own. Make your best decisions, but know that there are options.

When it comes to the health of yourself or the members of your family, you cannot leave it solely to anyone else. I am not in the medical field; I am not a member of the scientific world. I am just a mom, wife, career woman, sister, and daughter – nothing more. But I have learned some hard lessons about health and food allergies, and the lessons continue. I have also learned the hard way on how one person's allergies may impact the entire family. Some of the best medical and scientific minds exist in the world today, yet they only generalize when it comes to a family's health and well-being. You Specialize. **IT'S YOUR HEALTH-OWN IT**.

Throughout this book, I will mention different products. I'm not promoting anything; I am only identifying what worked for us. You make your own decisions, based on your own successes. And find what works best for you. I did substantial research and investigated the long-term potential side effects, while using each product judiciously, and found my family's successes by using the products that I identified.

Fewer things are more humbling, than for an adult to be giving the care and responsibility of a child. When that child is a newborn baby, the humility is even greater. But when that child is plagued with illness, you learn some cold hard facts, and you learn them quickly. You learn that nothing is more important to a good parent than ensuring the well-being of your little trooper. And you learn to forget your own self-centered and narcissistic moments, for the more important needs of the child. This is what good parents do, and I feel that I am no different. I'm not a doctor, scientist, or anyone associated with the medical field. I'm just a mother whose son was born with some of the most severe examples of how allergies are nothing to take for granted. And I want to tell you our story.

At the end of this book, an area has been established for your <u>note-taking</u> convenience. It will give the user a place to make annotations for referencing possible Food Allergies you may have experienced; as well as to provide an area to put your own ideas on how to handle them.

CONTENTS

Chapter 1 *Meningitis Scare*

If a person lives for 100 years, only 18 of those years are considered childhood. For the average child, very few things register in their active mind besides being a kid and making the best of those 18 years of life. Unless the child has a serious medical issue, most children and their parents don't sweat the little aches and pains; we just roll right through them. But if I knew then what I know now, some of the little aches and pains of my own childhood would have been big red flags for my Food Allergies and the ones that I would pass on to my son.

My awareness of Food Allergies did not become the 'Red Flag' until I went to my doctor one day, sometime back in the early part of 1990. I was in my 30s, and I thought that I was dying. I had researched my symptoms and come to the conclusion that I had a severe case of Meningitis (or so I had 'ass-u-me-d'). But I needed to see a doctor in order to confirm my findings. You know the saying, "Physician, heal thyself". There should be another one that states: "Patient, analyze thyself", because that is exactly what I did, but I was very, very wrong in my analysis.

After doing all my research, I was ready to follow Queen

Latifah and take a 'Last Holiday'. I was in so much pain, I believed that I was experiencing the classic symptoms of Meningitis: stiff neck (I could barely move it forward), respiratory distress (could barely breath without wheezing), fevers, night chills, night sweats, body and joint stiffness along with severe body aches, a deep, congested cough, mucus buildup in my sinuses and chest, nausea, vomiting, and severe head pains. I could barely get around, and thought that I was at the final stages. There is nothing more humbling to think you are dying, and then realize you're not. But I get ahead of myself.

I scheduled an appointment with my doctor, and my visit was a real eye-opener. After explaining to my doctor my diagnosis, I waited for his response. I'm thinking that I hit this diagnosis right on the head because I had every symptom described for Meningitis, but

Some Symptoms of Meningitis

∴ **High fever**
∴ **Stiff neck**
∴ **Stiff or sore muscles**
∴ **Stiff or sore joints**
∴ **Sensitivity to light**
∴ **Drowsiness**
∴ **Feeling of lethargy**
∴ **Nausea and/or vomiting**
∴ **Loss of appetite**
Some are difficult to observe in infants

evidently I missed one big symptom, and the doctor was more than happy to enlighten me. Giving me the look that said, "I am the doctor and you are not", his response was that I would not have been able to walk into his office if I had the final stages, or any stage of Meningitis. Not only did I walk in, but I drove myself to the appointment. The doctor actually offered to do a spinal tap if I wanted one. Really??? I'm thinking that I'm dying and he's thinking that I'm an idiot. Okay, so maybe I was a bit off the mark, but my symptoms were classic Meningitis. As I left his office without a backwards glance, I thought long and hard of what he had stated. And after thinking about it, I concluded that maybe he wasn't a Quack after all. And maybe I over-analyzed a bit, but the symptoms were textbook Meningitis. I have a high threshold for pain, but, from what my doctor described, I still would have had to be transported by ambulance if I was suffering from any stage of Meningitis. So, if it's not Meningitis, then what? I went back to the library to do more research.

For a more precise and 'in your face'
description of Meningitis and its symptoms,
please take the time to check out the website
NATIONAL MENINGITIS ASSOCIATION
www.nmaus.org

If you do experience the symptoms mentioned above, don't make assumptions; see your doctor. If its allergies, then you may be referred have your doctor refer you to an allergist. But if it's actual Meningitis, your doctor will know what to do. **DON'T ASSUME!!**

After more extensive research and coming up with nothing solid, I thought about what I was doing and what I was eating. Since my diet was basically the same diet that I was raised on, I didn't think anything of its content. I couldn't find a common factor with my diet or with what I was doing, so I decided that I would begin with the simplest thing – diet - and then move on from there. The first thing that I did was write down the foods that I would eat for the next week or two, and I'd only consume the items that were on the list. The list was short and easy to track, and for two weeks, it was enough to cover my basic needs. My diet included water, eggs, rice, fish, chicken, green veggies, and nothing else. I ate just these items for about two weeks. One of the first things that registered to me was that I could breathe better because normally, during the night, my breathing would be rough and I would wake up full of congestion in my chest and in my sinus area. But this time I woke up uncongested, and my head didn't ache so much. Then there was this feeling that my neck had lots of movement. Another symptom that I had, but didn't associate with Meningitis, was Lockjaw. This particular problem started when I was very young. It started so early, that I thought it was a normal part of my existence. Well, that was the very first thing that disappeared. I performed the diet for two weeks, but all of the symptoms were gone before the end of the first week. It didn't register in my small mind until later in the diet modification that my version of Meningitis was GONE! What The???

At the end of the second week, I couldn't wait to get back into the foods that I eliminated. For two reasons: first, they were tasty, and second, they could possibly indicate the problem. I had to learn real fast about diet modifications, because the very first thing that I re-introduced into my diet had me in tears. There is nothing more devastating than to find out that the one food you loved the most, hated your guts – literally.

The beauty of an Elimination Diet is that you can go back to eating basic foods in your effort to help yourself. You don't need a doctor or nutritionist; just go back to the basic food staples for living – nothing fancy or exotic

Not one hour after I took that first drink of my refreshing glass of milk, my stomach was in knots and my head was aching so badly, I thought it would explode. The real indicator of how badly milk and I did not get along happened the next morning. Prior to my diet, every morning I would wake up to my jaws locked in place. I would have to massage them before I started my day, in order for them to relax and operate normally. Well, I had to start the massage process again, and knew immediately that milk and I did not get along. I stopped drinking milk. Thinking that ice cream was not just milk alone, I decided I should be able to consume it. WRONG!!! Ice cream was not as immediate an impact, but once I consumed it a couple of times, I knew that I could not continue. Ice cream was removed from my diet. The rest of the foods were okay, so I moved on.

Chapter 3 MY VERY OWN REALIZATION

It's My Health, so I should own it

Immediately after the diet experiment, it was time for my menstrual cycle to begin, and I was dreading it. My menstrual cycle began when I was age twelve. Prior to the menstrual phenomenon, I was a Perfect Attendance student. But after my cycle started, I would miss at least one day of school each month. My menstrual cycle always appeared like clockwork, running the same pattern prior to the bleeding. I would have severe cramping and migraines, to the point that I could barely move. Once the bleeding started, some of the stomach pain would ease, and the head pressure subsided, but I would bleed like my insides were tearing apart. As I became an adult, not only did I bleed heavily but I would pass large clots of tissue. During all of my cycles, I would bleed so heavily that I could only use menstrual pads, the Super Maxi Pads – the biggest ones available. And I would go through at least two large boxes each cycle. Each cycle lasted for a minimum of seven days, and then I was free again for the next 21 days.

I know you are probably asking yourself why I was not taken to a doctor for my ailments when I was a small child. The best way to explain it is that, we had no money. I was raised in the projects and we were dirt poor. The only time that we saw a doctor was when the free clinic was set up once a year, in the project's recreation center. We would get dental checks, basic physicals and immunizations, but there was no money for doctor's visits. So, if we did not appear to be on death's-door, we kept it movin'. Our basic needs were met and, even with living in the projects, childhood was good and mostly healthy.

I have four sisters, yet none of them suffered like I did. During my youth, even with four sisters, lots of female cousins, and my mom, certain things were not discussed. So, I had to work my way through my cycle alone. I was not able to ask those intimate questions that I needed answers for. With each pending cycle's approach, I would get myself prepared for the aches and pains. I am not a pill-taker, but Bayer® aspirin was always at the ready for the eventual onslaught of pain. As I fast forward to the 90's and after my elimination diet, this time there was no pain. There were no severe stomach cramping, backaches, or migraines. What in the world??? This hadn't happened in over two decades, not since I started my menstrual cycle. It was a part of my norm! I was actually expecting it; not wanting it, but expecting it. WOW!!! No pain, just five days of moderate to very light bleeding. Could it be? Was I cured??? After this phenomenon, I realized that I was going to be okay. I wasn't dying from Meningitis or anything else (other than my own stupidity). I was allergic to Dairy.

Because I now knew that a lot of my ailments were simply

contributed to some of the foods that I ate, the work was easier. Was it that simple? And why didn't my doctors tell me to look at my diet? That was when I knew that in order to get healthy and stay healthy, I could not rely solely on my doctor, because the responsibility for my health was in my hands. So I took charge. It's my health and I began to OWN IT.

Chapter 4   My Pregnancy and Allergies

Now that I am beginning to have some type of control over most of my health, I focused my energies on getting pregnant. A feat that was harder than I could imagine.

My husband and I were at it for over twelve years, with no results. I tried everything imaginable (and some things unimaginable), with no success. I was given all types of advice – from standing on my head to having sex during your menstrual cycle (??). Nothing worked. I was never going to get pregnant.

Then, low and behold and after over twelve years of trying everything possible to get pregnant, one of those little Olympic swimmers got through and latched onto an egg, holding on for dear life. Unfortunately, in my excitement of pregnancy, I forgot about my food issues. And by not following through with my pre-planned food restriction diet during pregnancy, I passed my severe food allergies to my son. And so the story truly begins.

GOD in his infinite wisdom knew how desperate I was for a child. Ever since I was a little one myself, I've always wanted children. I vowed that if I ever got married, I would have at least a half dozen 'rugrats'. But that was not to be. For over twelve years of marriage, I was unable to conceive. I tried everything, every trick, but nothing worked. And there were a lot of tricks to perform. (But that's an entirely different book).

When other women had birth control pills, I had pregnancy test kits. Once a month, I would take a test and once a month, I would be disappointed. But, one day, my nephew and I were out jogging and I could barely breathe. He suggested that I see a doctor to get it checked out and I stated that I would. It was also time for my monthly pregnancy test, so I decided to take the test before I made the appointment. This was the Friday before Father's Day, 1994. I took the test, expecting the same results. I was wrong. It came back positive. I thought that it was a bad kit. I always kept extra kits, so I was able to take the test two more times, and each test came back positive. I still could not believe what I am seeing, so I go to a walk- in clinic. The on-site doctor confirmed that I was in my very first month of pregnancy. "Congratulations!", she stated. Though I was in the very first month of the pregnancy, when I went to work that next Monday morning, I had on maternity clothes and sporting my biggest grin, ever.

My pregnancy was the best. I was hardly sick; no morning sickness; I ate well and was extremely energetic and happy. Forgoing my allergy issue, I forced myself to consume milk for the baby because of the calcium and protein benefits. The few times I was sick, it was because of the milk I drank. At work one day, I was talking in casual conversation with a friend of mine about how milk was making me ill, but that I needed it for the baby. He stated that I should stop drinking the milk if it was bothering my stomach, and try orange juice. He, also, enlightened me on the availability of orange juices that were fortified with calcium, and suggested I try it. I did, and it was the second best advice I got during my pregnancy, because not only did the pains go away, but my baby seemed to like it. He was always moving around, but would calm down when I drank the juice. After that, pregnancy was easy. I slept good, ate well (without over eating), and continued my daily activities without any problems. But no one could prepare me for what would happen when my 'water broke'.

The day I was to give birth, I cleaned my entire house, took a nice warm bath, and got into bed around midnight. Less than an hour later, my water broke and everything went downhill from there.

I was scheduled to be in a birthing room and I was supposed to have my son as naturally as possible. That never happened. That little human being did not want to come down. I leaked water from after midnight until my son was removed, via C-section at 9:04pm that night. Through the entire process, I was in a lot of pain, but only did a little bit of complaining. Even when I was in pain, I was smiling, because I knew that my baby was on his way. At least that was what I thought. Little did I know that my baby was dying, and not only could he have died, but so could I.

The on-site doctor was supposed to have been the best in the field, but his bedside manner was the worst. I was keeping him from his golf appointment by delaying the delivery, so he attempted to help expedite the process by 'snipping' me a bit, to help me dilate. Since I was leaking lots of water after my water broke, the doctor's lack of patience only made the water gush harder and flow faster. And since he was dressed in street clothes and not doctor's scrubs, his clothes got wet from the rush of water. Served him right, but, unfortunately for me, he never returned. So I sat there for hours without a doctor. I had great nurses, though. One nurse in particular saved my son's life. Nurse Mary was able to prove to the next doctor that the umbilical cord was wrapped around my son's neck, which saved both our lives.

Eventually, after the issue with the doctor and my water flow, a few hours later I finally received a visit from the evening shift doctor. By then, my mom was about to call down the law on the entire hospital staff, due to neglect. I didn't complain but she sure did. She very impolitely (using very creative cursing) informed the doctor that I was in excruciating pain, and for them to give me something for it. Eventually I was given an epidural. After that, the pain subsided but only on one side of my body. The anesthesiologist and the on-site doctor didn't believe me, and the nurse was a little bit skeptical. But, with modern medicine and some sort of monitoring process, the nurse was able to prove that I was still in pain. Whenever I stated that I was having severe pain, the monitor indicated a problem. Well, before it was over, the anesthesiologist was sweating bullets and I was given another epidural shot for the pain. Finally, I was not in pain, but I still had only dilated less than one centimeter.

Just on a whim, the nurse decided to place a monitor on the baby to check his pulse rate whenever I had a contraction. After a couple of contractions, she got the doctor to observe, stating that she believed that the umbilical cord was wrapped around the baby's neck and I would need to go in for surgery, immediately. My personal doctor, who had just returned from a vacation not two hours prior, was contacted. He informed them to prep the room and he would be there within a couple of minutes. I was moved to the operating room at 9:00 PM and my son was pulled out at 9:04 PM, via C-section. I was blessed with a 9 pound, 2 ounce, healthy baby boy, with a baritone cry. During the entire process, I was wide awake and alert and grinning from ear-to-ear. My baby was coming and I could not have been happier. But that was not the end, only the beginning.

During my pregnancy, I attended a wedding. And during that wedding, I had a conversation with a cousin to my sister-in-law. I was telling her that because of my age, my doctor suggested that I may consider Amniocentesis. Amniocentesis is a medical procedure used in prenatal diagnosis of chromosomal abnormalities. The process requires the removal of a small amount of the amniotic fluid from the sac around the baby in the womb. It has its benefits, but it has its complications as well. The person that I was having the discussion with asked me one simple question: "Then what?" At first I was a bit lost, so I asked her to explain. She simply stated that if I had the amniocentesis, then what would I do? Would I abort my child or would I keep it? That question put it all into perspective for me. There was no way I would have this test, because the bottom line was that regardless of the outcome, I would keep my child. The next day, I contacted my doctor's office to cancel that appointment. The test was long forgotten.

On the day of his birth and as I looked into the eyes of my hour-old son, I was glad that I did not jeopardize his birth with the test. My son was a healthy, strapping boy – or at least I thought so, until he needed to be fed.

Per **WIKIPEDIA.ORG -** *Amniocentesis (also referred to as* **amniotic fluid test or AFT**) *is a medical procedure used in prenatal diagnosis of chromosomal abnormalities and fetal infections, and also used for sex determination in which a small amount of amniotic fluid, which contains fetal tissues, is sampled from the amniotic sac surrounding a developing fetus, and the fetal DNA is examined for genetic abnormalities.* *Per*

MARCHOFDIMES.ORG- **Amniocentesis** *(also called amnio) is a common prenatal test used to diagnose certain birth defects and genetic conditions. Genetic conditions are health conditions and birth defects that are passed down to a baby from mom and dad. BE AWARE – AN AMNIOCENTESIS COMES WITH RISKS refer to www.mayoclinic.org to find out more*

Chapter 5   And So His Story Begins

One of my plans for my son was to breastfeed him. I was really into the process, so when it was time for his first feeding, I was so excited and couldn't wait. We were going to bond. Or not. The reality of breastfeeding was not the fantasy I envisioned. It was a nightmare for the both of us. As soon as I put him to my breast, he screamed. Not cry, but scream. And then he did the unthinkable: he bit me! He bit me so hard that I had to pry his little 'gums' apart to get my nipple out. He screamed, I moaned, and we were both in tears by the time the nurse returned. When I told the nurse of what had happen, she was not convinced. She stated that babies don't have teeth and can't bite. I told her that this one did and he bit me, hard. Those little gums were sharp as razor blades. She tried to assist with the next attempt, but my son was not having it. There's nothing like contorting your breast to fit between a baby's locked gums. Not gonna happen. He refused to open his little mouth and had the hardest look on his face: the look of pain. I informed the nurse that this was not working and my baby was going to starve. She suggested that I try what was considered to be the next best thing to mother's milk, a Soy milk formula. He was very content with this, and that was what we went home with. My son and I were going home, and I couldn't wait to get him there.

The first two weeks of being at home were both a joy and a nightmare. Not because of the usual, but the unusual. I had a closet full of Pampers and they were gone within the first two weeks of bringing my baby home. He would drink his formula and immediately produce liquid stools. His feedings were not staying in his body long enough for him to sustain and gain any nutritional value. It was like his mouth was directly attached to his rectal area, bypassing all digestive system organs and functions. The poor thing was having constant, and painful, stools. His digestive system did not give the formula time to process before it literally ripped through his little body. If he wasn't pooping it out, he was throwing it up.

As a matter of fact, I recall one particular diaper changing episode, vividly. My son was not sleeping completely through the night, so whenever he was asleep, I attempted to not disturb him. This particular night, he wasn't sleeping well. His stools were runny all day and throughout the night. Most of the time, he would awaken when I changed his diaper, but this time I had a brilliant plan. Since I was sleeping in his bedroom that night, I was able to hear (and smell) everything a lot better. I was awaken by a strong baby poopy smell and knew that I needed to change his diaper, but didn't want to disturb his beauty sleep. As the creative mother that I am, I decided to change his diaper while he was still asleep in his crib. You know, don't awaken the sleeping giant. It was definitely the wrong move, people. The room was lit by a small lamp, so the lighting was not the best for viewing, only sleeping. As I wiped clean my little poopy son's bottom, I needed to get closer to ensure that I had done a thorough job. Mothers of the world please don't do this. It's not a smart move, at all. As I got close enough to see if my cleaning efforts were successful, his little butt cheeks began to quiver. I'm pretty sure that most people have heard the statement, 'Fire in the Hole!'. Well, you cannot appreciate it more than when a baby's bottom is about to blow. My goodness! I was able to jerk my head away just in time because, even in his deepest sleep, his aim was true. His butt cheeks quivered and out shot a stream of liquid stool that blew where my head had been. I know some people believe that a baby's wet diaper is good for the complexion, but I can't believe that baby poop works as a facial mask. I almost found out first hand.

After that night, I was very cautious of the cleaning processes and rear ends. But the diarrhea went on for the first two weeks of his life and then the tide turned, negatively. My son was bleeding in his stool.

That night, my husband and I rushed him to the emergency room. I was so upset that I couldn't talk and had to write down what was going on. On that night and with Blessings from above, the on-staff pediatrician was a pediatric oncologist. The first thing he said to me was that the problem was not what I thought it was. I guess, by looking at my distressed face, he assumed that I thought he was dying. I did. But he confirmed by running some tests, that I was wrong. He simply stated that our baby was experiencing what is called a Fissure Tear in his rectal area. I'm looking at the doctor as if I knew what that was, but I didn't have a clue. All I heard was 'He's not dying'.

The fissure tear was caused by the many painful bowel movements and the intermittent hard stools that my son was experiencing. Even though most of his stools were runny, he was straining a lot to pass them through. So when he experienced any type of stool, he was straining harder than was normal for a baby, and the straining generated the tear of tissue in the anal area of the rectum. The doctor informed us that the tear would heal. He sent us home with one piece of advice: Change his baby formula. Immediately I did, and the results were fast. By the way, straining is not good for anyone's blood pressure.

The very next day, my son's stools stabilized. They were solid and not so frequent. He was enjoying the newer formula and I was enjoying the new peace of mind. But they say to take your wins where you can, and I understand why. This newest win did not last long, and that became the pattern.

I believe that we tried every formula on the shelf, and every formula created its own unique problem for my baby. I'm not so sure I would have even noticed the problems if I'd been a very young mom, but I hope that I would have, because my baby suffered through his first two years of life so badly to the point that I didn't know if he would survive.

As I mentioned before, each new formula created a different medical problem for my baby. The next formula after the Soy-based product was identified as the next best thing after Soy. It was, for one moment, but it also presented a new problem: the dreaded "C" word, Colic.

Nothing will keep a baby (and parent) up like a bout with colic. The pain is excruciating for both child and parent. My baby's little gut knots up and the cramps are like torture to them. The screams were enough to make you pull out your hair. This would go on for days, and always at the same time of day. It was very bizarre. My first and (unfortunately) my only child, and he stayed miserable. We were back at the grocery store looking for a new formula.

Every formula states that it's the best, so it was difficult to decide which one was truly the best to use. I took the approach of believing that the most expensive one should be the best. Wrong!!! You haven't seen anything until you have observed your baby do a 'Linda Blair-Exorcist' number with vomiting. That projectile vomiting is a sight to behold, especially from something so small.

One of the most precious gifts that I received at my baby shower was a couple of packages of 100% American-made, cotton baby diapers and Onesies. The diapers made the best cloths for catching anything 'baby wet' and the Onesies were easier to change. When the vomiting started, the liquids went everywhere, and those diapers were a blessing. I feel that they are a necessity when having little ones around. The cloths absorb well, clean up easily in the wash, and last for a long time.

The projectile vomiting went on for days, and the stools were more frequent, but not watery. It was almost as if to smell the formula, would trigger a reaction. One of the problems that existed with each formula was my baby's inability to breathe, uncongested. Whenever he would be in bed, he would snore, a wet, congested-type of snoring. I know they say that babies hardly sleep at night, but my son's sleeping pattern was a long ways off the norm. He would sleep in snatches; a little here, a little there, because he could hardly breathe. So when he would sleep quietly, I would get nervous. And I had a valid reason to feel this way because, twice, before the age of six months, our son stopped breathing in his sleep. And that's a terrifying thing to experience.

The first time, he was no more than a month and a half. Because he was so new and miraculous to me, I rarely let him sleep without constantly checking, every few minutes. Yeah, I know I was a bit anal, but it paid off. On one of those occasions, I noticed that his breathing was very quiet; a little too quiet. Normally, whenever my son would sleep, he would snore, and his chest would rattle with congestion. Even at his quietest sleep state, there would still be a light snoring. So I gave him a little touch to see if he would respond. Nothing. I gently turned him over and lightly ran my finger across his nose. Nothing! I picked him up and put my ear to his little chest. Nothing!!! His little lips were turning blue and I panicked. I took him to my husband, telling him not to let my baby die. He gave him mouth-to-mouth and nose breaths, and then he gave him a 'baby' Heimlich pat on the back, and resuscitated our son back to life. His first response was to cough up mucus, and then he started to scream. I never cried so hard before. He was okay. The rest of that day and night, I watched him sleep, listening for any changes to his breathing pattern. After that episode, if his breathing changed from congestive to quiet, I would awaken him from his sleep. Strangely enough, this happened more times than not. But that was my first experience with what I believe to be Sudden Infant Death Syndrome (SIDS). SIDS is a parent's worst nightmare. I read all the books, and tried all of the positions and bedding suggested, but nothing worked. None of the positions or bedding prepared me for the fact that a baby's bronchial tube is no match for thick mucus buildup. Babies have no idea on how to cough up the mucus. When those little tubes get clogged, the air will not pass but, as a parent, what do you know, and what can you do. After the second episode, which I was able to handle myself, I watched him closely. One of the things that I did, during this close observation period, was to stop giving my son formula when putting him to sleep. Before any extended naps or attempted nighttime sleeping, I gave him a bottle of warm water, with nothing in it. This helped tremendously. It forced up lots of mucus and his snoring wasn't as congested. He wasn't happy at first with the water, but he easily adapted to it. I also learned how to 'pat' a baby's back to loosen up the phlegm and keep the mucus moving.

And after the bout with the expensive formula and the SIDS, My son and I went back to the grocery store, to a new formula and a new episode. I expected no less.

More information can be found relating to SIDS (Sudden Infant Death Syndrome) on the following websites:
Center for Disease Control www.cdc.gov/sids
American SIDS Institute www.sids.org

Chapter 6 Did I Miss any Allergies?
Can't see how, because it looks like he had all of them

By the time our son was six months old, he had experienced every dietary allergic reaction known. Some symptoms were common to all. For instance, he would break out in little bumps and his skin would be as rough as sandpaper. I spent a fortune on creams, lotions, and oils with no success. He would also experience severe episodes of Cradle Cap and Thrush.

Cradle Cap is a yellowish crusty, scaly, patchy skin rash that appears on the baby's scalp. It is also called Seborrhea Dermatitis. For the cradle cap, I was told by his pediatrician, to use a very harsh shampoo which contained coal tar. It was too harsh. The shampoo stripped his hair of natural oils but did nothing for the cradle cap.

Cradle Cap and Thrush are both signs of a yeast infection, allergy-triggered

And as for the thrush, I was told to wipe his tongue off with a clean wash cloth and just keep an eye out. Thrush is a fungal infection in the mouth, also known as Candida Fungus or Yeast. What I experienced with my son was that the fungus would occur in other areas of the body, as well as the mouth. There were samples of the fungus that would occur in the folds of the skin, such as in his armpits or around the neck. There were even signs of the fungus located in his diaper area, triggering diaper rashes. I tried the diaper rash creams and the special 'sensitive for baby's skin' soaps, oils, and lotions. Nothing worked, and I found that the baby oil made things worse. None of the issues went away, so I had to find alternatives to dealing with them all.

I did some research to get a better understanding of what I was dealing with. My son and I spent a lot of time in the library, one of my favorite places to be still today. We also spent hours wandering around grocery stores. We really spent a lot of hours at one particular grocery store. During that time, I couldn't find anything that would work for my baby at any of the other grocery stores that I shopped. At the store called Fresh Fields, I would read labels and check prices. Store managers probably thought that I was casing the joint with my baby as an alibi, because I didn't buy anything for a long time. After gathering the information that I needed, I would go home and do more research. Once I got my notes organized, I developed a shopping list and headed back to the Fresh Fields Market, in Wheaton, Illinois. This store was not close to my home, so the trip had to be well planned. My budget was limited, so I had to ensure that what I purchased was what we needed. The store was not cheap, but the items that I needed were only available for me at this particular store. This was during the

'90's. I purchased Jojoba oil, baby formula, and Dr. Bronner's®
Unscented Baby-mild Liquid Soap. Then I went back home to test
things out.

For his cradle cap, I used a baby wash cloth, and slowly but
very lightly, I would rub Jojoba oil on his scalp. This would help to
loosen the caking effect of the cradle cap, and it was very effective.

To remove the crusty residue, I bathed him and washed his hair with
Dr. Bronner's® Unscented Baby-mild Liquid Soap. Add a very tiny
amount of Tea Tree Oil to the Soap for that extra boost, if needed.
Not only did it remove the patchy cradle cap residue, but it was very
effective in removing signs of Thrush in other areas of the body.

For the thrush in his mouth, I cleaned the tongue and insides
of the mouth with a very sterile washcloth. Afterwards, I would
have him drinking only water before lying down to sleep.

I was able to control the cradle cap and thrush, but the
congestion would not go away. The vomiting was severe some days,
and mild other days, but it was always there. By the time he was nine
months old, my son experienced three episodes of Pneumonia, had
gone through every formula on the shelf including the ones from
Fresh Market, and he was still very congested and he slept, miserably.
At that point, I'd had enough. There is no way that one baby should

go through this much just to eat. Through all of this, there was one common denominator: baby's milk. My son experienced his last bout of pneumonia while at the pediatrician's office. I stated that my son was allergic to dairy and that there is no way a child should react to every formula in a similar manner. His doctor made one statement that has stayed with me all of this time – "I'm a doctor and I Generalize with the patient. You are a parent and you Specialize." She also agreed with my conclusion but stated that, although he demonstrated signs of allergic response, Brandon would have to stay on formula until he was one-year's old. She also directed me to take him to an allergy specialist to be tested, which I did. Trust me when I say that the story does not end here. It was only the beginning.

Chapter 7   The Allergy Test?

Most babies at nine months' of age are as carefree, and as happy as can be. As a parent, it can be a nightmare to watch a baby taking an allergy test.

At the allergy specialist's office, the nurses treated my son with great care. I was told that he was the youngest person to ever get tested in their office. They were very nurturing. But, no matter how much care you give a patient, there are things that very few are prepared to deal with, and those can strike right at the core of the mother instinct of a nurse.

The first test required that fifteen small dots be placed on my son's back. He was to lie on his stomach, so they gave him a book to look at. As the dots were placed equidistant apart, an 'essential' oil droplet was placed on each dot. Each oil represented a food-allergy trigger that included oils for shellfish, oats, dairy, soy, egg, nuts, etc. There was a time period to wait for results, in order to identify the allergic trigger. Well, that didn't happen. Not long into the test, whelps begin to appear on his back and he starting scratching the affected areas. To calm his reaction, a nurse offered two items. One was an adrenaline shot and the other was a dose of Actifed®. I asked what the difference was, and was told that there was very little difference.

Since, during that time, I could purchase the Actifed® over–the-counter, I chose that for my son. Actifed® worked immediately. The reaction wasn't as bad as it could have been, but the whelps merged together, making it difficult to identify all of the essences that he was allergic to. There were at least four allergens that were readily, identifiable from the test – Soy,

Certain medicines may be readily available, over-the-counter, but should not be administered to your child until you have consulted with your pediatric advisor. Even the mildest of medications can have a detrimental effect.

Dairy, Oats, and Shellfish. Interestingly enough, the first two had already been identified.

To complete his testing, we were required to return, on a different day to test the airborne allergens. That particular test did not go real well, at all.

The dots for this test were run up and down his arms, so as not to further irritate the histamines from the previous test. Almost immediately, he began to scratch, but this time his eyes started to water, his sinuses started draining, and he started coughing with congestion. It was driving him crazy. Immediately, he was given an injection of adrenaline to calm the histamine reaction. It took a few minutes before he was able to calm down. The coughing did not subside because the congestive reaction caused a buildup of mucus in his chest. The allergist stated his reaction was not something that was caused by his testing, and he could not be held accountable. I left his office, immediately.

Luck has it that my son had a pediatric appointment an hour after the allergy testing. So we went directly to the appointment. When we arrived, seeing how difficult it was for my son to breathe, his pediatrician immediately started him on a breathing treatment, followed by a steroid treatment. Once the treatments were started, I was asked to explain what had happened, which I did.

His pediatrician was very unhappy and stated that it would not be in our best interest to take my son back to that allergist. I knew that I would not. The one good thing that happened during the appointment was that he was given a prescription for an Epipen®. Epipen is a prescription epinephrine (adrenaline) auto-injector, for personal use. At nine months of age, my son had an emergency adrenaline dispenser. I had asked the allergist the question, "What if he has a reaction every day? What am I supposed to do?" His response was what I thought it would be. "Give him an injection every time he reacts." And he stated this with confidence. Really? Every day? That was not going to happen. Again, I went back to the library to do extensive research. In the '90s, we lived in Naperville, Illinois, and that city had a very good library system, available to the public. And it was within walking distance to my home. My son and I were regular users of the library's research materials.

Once I explained to his pediatrician what had happened, she politely informed me that I could take him home, but that would not be a sound move. He was having difficulty breathing, and needed a confined and controlled environment to stabilize his respiration. She stated that he needed to be put in the hospital, and I agreed. Let me tell you, in the first four years of my son's life, it felt like we spent more time in the hospital than out.

My son received his first EPIPEN® at the tender age of nine months but as of today, he has not been administered any doses. You have to renew your prescription, yearly, and the cost is skyrocketing.
[Supply + Demand = price gouging]
My son's first PEN was less than $18, and his most current PEN cost $474, before insurance

---

Chapter 8   PDR-Physician's Desk Reference

My son was also placed on all sorts of medicines to help him breath. We were sent home from the hospital with so many prescriptions, it boggled the mind. I was told by his pediatrician that he would be on his medications for the rest of his life. I had to purchase a breathing machine for inhaling some of the medication, and he was given prescriptions for Prednisone®, Albuterol®, Intal®, and some over- the-counter medications were suggested, as well. Prednisone® is a synthetic corticosteroid used to treat allergic reactions. Albuterol® is a bronchodilator that relaxes muscles in the lungs and increases air flow to the lungs. Intal® is a prescription drug for the treatment of asthma. I went back to the library to research the medications.

One of the things that I came across during my research was references to the Physician's Desk Reference Books. I also recall one of my son's many pediatricians referring to a huge tome for guidance. When I asked him what it was, he said that it was the Physician's Desk Reference book. The doctor's edition was unabridged, and that was the reason for its large size. I'm thinking to myself that it would be a great help to a parent for at-home use, not realizing that I would one day get lucky. That day came sooner than expected.

While walking around the grocery store, I came across the

book area. How fortunate it was for me, that one paperback book stood out like a neon light? On the cover of this book were the words PHYSICIAN'S DESK REFERENCE (PDR), and priced for only $7.99. Can you believe the luck! We had our very own PDR for home use. That book was and still is a true blessing because, whenever I get a prescription, I am able to evaluate the content and possible side effects before administering it to my son. It was beneficial for me and my husband, as well.

One of the statements that his pediatrician made was that he would be on the medications for the rest of his life. That is, hopefully, a very long time, but I was not in agreement with her statement. It didn't make sense that a child should be continuously subjected to so much mind and mood altering prescription drugs. I was directed to follow the usage guidelines. That wasn't going to happen, either.

The first thing I did, with the help of my PDR, was to evaluate the side effects of each medication and the medications' benefits. I was extremely cautious with the Prednisone®. Its short-term effects were, let's say, effective, but the long-term effects were counter-effective. I knew that he needed this product, so I modified the handling processes. Instead of taking the prescribed dose, I changed the dosage by half at each dose. For example, if the Prednisone® prescription stated to take two pills, four times per day, I would give my son the exact dose initially prescribed, for the first day. On the second day, I would give him one pill, four times per day; one pill, twice per day; then finally one pill for the last day. By the end of the second day, his breathing would have stabilized and the medication's half-life effect would continue to work. This helped to minimize the long-term negative side effects of the steroids. And there were quite a few negatives. Prednisone®, for short-term relief, is extremely effective for respiratory distress. The systemic effect from a breathing treatment, for Albuterol is immediate, as well. The combination of the two drugs can be the first line of defense for respiratory distress, as well as in calming the histamine reactors to allergies. We did not use the prescribed Intal because it contained a product that was an allergic trigger for my son. Another product that became a staple in our home was Actifed®. We kept on hand this over-the-counter medication because it contained the same active ingredient that was contained in an adrenaline shot. And, I would find out later that it was just as effective. Actifed® is an effective pseudoephedrine histamine-blocker and decongestant. With the doctors prescribing so much medication and my son struggling with allergic triggers, I had to find a way to keep him healthy and safe, while protecting him from drug interactions and reactions. I had my work cut out for me, but it would be worth it in the long run.

Chapter 9   a Year and a Day

As I mentioned earlier, per his pediatrician's directive, my son would have to remain on formula until he was at least one year's of age, regardless of his allergic response to dairy. As soon as he turned a year and a day, he was put through withdrawal. I took away his milk bottle and pacifier. What the heck was I thinking, or was I thinking at all, because that was one of the roughest days of both our lives. But we made it through. On that day, my son stopped drinking baby formula, and started drinking Rice Dream® Rice Drink, which he still drinks today. Not only did my son like Rice Drink, but the drink liked him back. No problems. And because I started him on Rice Milk at an early age, he will not drink any other milk substitute. For him, this is milk. And for me, it was a life saver. It contains as much Calcium and Vitamin D as milk. The only limitation is the amount of protein, but we can get protein from other sources.

I came across Rice Dream® Rice Drink during one of our trips to Fresh Fields, a Whole Foods Market division in Naperville, Illinois. At the time, I thought that the price was a bit steep, but once we started using it, I realized that it was more than worth the money. It easily paid for itself in peace of mind and doctor's visit reductions. Well worth the money. But the biggest benefit was in my son's sleeping. Prior to the introduction of the Rice Drink, whenever my son would sleep he would snore. His snoring was a rattling, wet snore. After about six months on the Rice Milk, I was able to sleep at night because my son was finally sleeping. It took that long for me to believe that he was actually sleeping and hadn't stopped breathing. There were a few episodes during his second year of life, but none were related to Dairy consumption. However, I'm about to learn some hard lessons about hidden allergy triggers, and they will not be pretty.

I'm thinking that we have finally gotten control of a serious allergy problem. It was a rough first year but we made it. From here on out, everything else would be a piece of cake. Yeah, right. Wishful thinking on my part. The hardest part of the entire process was watching my son struggle, but he was a trooper. Rarely did he let any of this get him down. But his momma was having the toughest of times. While I worked to keep my son healthy, I neglected my own health. And I would pay dearly for this.

Eventually I was pregnant again. I was very excited and couldn't wait for the new arrival. My son needed a playmate. But that was not to be. A couple of months into my second pregnancy, I was required to attend training. My mom went with me and my son, to babysit while I trained. Within two days of the training and very early on a Friday morning, I started to bleed and pass massive blood clots. I cleaned myself up and got ready to go to my class. After about two hours in the training, I excused myself to go to the school's clinic. I informed them of my problem, asked for something to help me through the day, and then I returned to class. At the end of the class day, I returned to my hotel room, and prepared my mom and son for a trip to North Carolina. There, they would stay until my training was completed. In my misery, I was unable to focus on anything. I'd had a miscarriage. I knew that my parents would take good care of my son while I got myself together. It was a long three months separation from my miracle baby, but it was needed.

There are a number of good dairy substitutes for children with dairy allergies. Shop around but be mindful of the facts that some dairy substitutions can trigger reactions, if allergic.

Chapter 10 Peanut Butter
What next – AIR???

On a day that I was not feeling so well, I kept my son home with me. I didn't have the energy to take him to the sitter's, but had not realized that I didn't have the energy to entertain him, either. Though I was sick and exhausted, my son was not. There's nothing like a very active toddler being around you, when you can barely lift your head up to observe them.

My son walked everywhere in the house, baby talking his little head off. All I could do was watch and hope that I could keep my eyes open and my hearing alert. After a few hours of baby babble and toddler toddling, I decided that I would try something to kind of tone down the babbling, at least. Couldn't do anything about the walking but I could work on the baby talking.

Well, at a year and a half, my son was eating better, and I thought that his allergies were under control. So, on one of my sickest days, I was not prepared for what would happen next.

I remember watching my mom stick a spoon full of peanut

butter in one of my nieces' mouth, in an attempt to get her to quiet down. It worked, at least for her. She quieted and began to chew, trying to dislodge the clump of peanut butter that had her mouth stuck shut. Well, don't try this at home, because I did, and paid dearly for it.

As my son came around the corner for the Umpteenth time, I attempted to stick a spoon of peanut butter in his mouth. Let me tell you, that little boy had some quick reflexes, because he clamped his mouth shut before the spoon could reach it. It was as if he could smell it coming. Then he screamed, that loud, ear-piercing, bone-chilling scream; then he clamped his lips tighter and rubbed the peanut butter up the side of his face and around his neck with his wrist, and walked away, but returned a few minutes later. And let me tell you, if I could have beaten myself that day, I would have. To see the damage that I put my son through was enough to break me of my melancholy and get it together. That little boy was a hot mess.

He wasn't crying or upset, but he looked as if he had been beaten, badly. Here we go again. My son was allergic to peanut butter. My Goodness!!! What else could go wrong? Do not ask yourself a question like that, you may not like the answer. My answer came later, but for now, I have to deal with the newest allergy: Peanut Butter.

Luck has it, I always had either Actifed® or Sudafed® available, and so I gave him a dose of the Actifed®. Actifed® is a registered trademark for a combination antihistamine and nasal decongestant that was suggested at the time, for children with severe cold and flu-like systems. Sudafed® is the brand name and registered trademark for an over-the-counter decongestant. Both contain the ingredient - Pseudoephedrine (a decongestant used to shrink blood vessels in the nasal cavity) but at the time, Actifed® contained an antihistamine, as well, which blocks histamine receptors from triggering allergic reactions. It did not take long to work, and I was very happy and fortunate, because if he had ingested the peanut butter, he could have gone into Anaphylactic Shock. Anaphylactic Shock is an immediate allergic reaction, causing serious bodily stress such as rash, hives, itchy, respiratory distress, or even death. My son's initial response to the Peanut butter was similar to receiving a severe burn. The response that he had was also similar to the response he had in the hospital when I tried to breastfeed him. The scream was excruciating and the reaction immediate. The difference was, with the Peanut butter, every place that he wiped with his wrist, was covered with whelps. His eyes watered and his nose was runny. He was not wheezing because he did not ingest any of the peanut butter, but he was congested. All of these symptoms subsided within an hour of taking the Actifed®, but it was a near miss.

Chapter 11 D&C

As I mentioned earlier, I was not feeling well but my son was more important. I was not feeling well because the day before, I had had a D&C after another miscarriage. Only a month earlier, my doctor confirmed that I was pregnant but the pregnancy would not go full term. I was experiencing what was called 'Beta' Strep. You ask yourself, "What is Beta Strep?" That was the same thing that I was rolling over in my mind, when my doctor said it. As my doctor talked on, all I could think of was that there was so much stuff about babies and pregnancy that no one tells you. As to the question, Beta Strep (Strep B) is a bacterium that may be found in a woman's vagina or rectum area. In pregnant women, it can be passed to the baby. If not diagnosed in time, it may cause the newborn to suffer meningitis, sepsis, pneumonia, and even stillborn. For the mother, it may trigger pre-mature labor or rupture of the membrane before 37 weeks, fever during labor, urinary tract infection, and or rupture of membrane up to 18 hours before delivery. It was another one of those 'Deer in the Headlights' moment. There was no way that I could disregard my doctor's information because she was the best there was, but I could not accept it. Even with the Ultrasound showing that there was nothing in the 'Sac', I still refuse to believe that I would miscarry, again; but it happened and this time, it was worse than before. I lost so much blood and bled so heavily for two weeks that I had to have a D&C. I was devastated. D&C or Dilation and Curettage is a procedure to remove tissue from your womb, after a miscarriage. It is the widening of the cervix and the surgical removal of part of the lining. It may also be performed because of spotting between periods, or to remove tissue that may cause heavy or irregular periods (menstrual cycle). My issue was nothing compared to my son's. I would live but he may not have.

Fortunately, he was okay, but I was not. I would find out later that my 'Beta Strep' infection was so severe that it was causing me complications. My uterus was so enlarged that it was comparably three times the normal size. I would need a hysterectomy. What next?

Chapter 12   What about Me?

At this point in my life, I am starting to realize that I need to take charge of my health. While I was doing everything possible to keep my little man healthy, I forgot all about his momma. My son was about six months old when I developed Strep Throat (Strep A). I had never before experienced this, and believe that due to the new mother stress, my immunities were very low. Though my immunities were low, I felt that I would only need 24 hours to get myself together, so that I could get back to taking care of everybody else. Well, unfortunately, while wearing that Super Woman cape, it got caught up on the hook of life. I could not do it all: the working outside of the home, and working rotating shifts, taking physical care of the home, and cooking almost every meal, taking care of a newborn, taking care of two teenage boys, and taking care of my husband. I thought that I could do it all, but at close to 40 years of age, something had to give, and what gave was ME. I was running myself into the grave, but, even when I got Strep Throat, I still would not acknowledge this. Not until my doctor diagnosed me with Beta Strep a year later did I realize that there was a problem. But the true reality of my health and its poor state was after the first miscarriage following my son's birth. During a follow-up visit with my doctor, I was required to take some tests. The testing brought everything into, perspective. I was informed that I could no longer have any babies and if I attempted to do so, it would be my last. My uterus was so enlarged and infected that it needed to be removed. I needed a hysterectomy.

I was in denial and refused to have it done. I became pregnant again. This time, even though the doctor's test indicated that I was positive for pregnancy; further tests proved that there was nothing inside of the egg. No embryo, no fetus, just an empty shell. I was also informed that I could have a surgical miscarriage (D&C). I refused, in hopes that my doctor was wrong and I was right. The doctor won out, because within the next two weeks, I miscarried. As I mentioned before, the miscarriage was so hard and heavy, it was the sickest that I had ever been. My son brought me back to reality that day, with his reaction to Peanut butter. I had a somewhat healthy baby boy, so I figured, be happy and content with the Blessings.

After the drama of the PEANUT BUTTER day, and the disaster of my miscarriage, I scheduled a follow-up appointment with my doctor to discuss options. I had no options; my only choice was a hysterectomy. The operation was scheduled. I was to have a partial hysterectomy. I would retain my ovaries.

On the day of the surgery, and as I waited for the doctor to prep, I was informed that I would have a total hysterectomy, removing all ovaries, as well. And that Mesh would also be used to eliminate the development of scar tissue. Before the surgery, I needed to have a discussion with my doctor because this was not what we had discussed. My doctor looked me in my eyes, and asked if I needed my ovaries, that she felt that I didn't want another surgery later on to remove then. Once should be enough. Because my doctor was one of the best in the field, and I knew she had my interest at heart, I agreed. I would receive a total hysterectomy.

After waking up from the surgery, the first thing that I noticed was a small patch on my right hip. Asking the doctor what the patch was, she told me it was a Hormone Replacement Therapy Patch (HRT). HRT is given to some women whose estrogen and progesterone levels drop significantly because of menopause. HRT tops up a woman's levels of essential hormones. It replaces the hormones that are no longer being produced, after a woman goes through menopause. I stated I did not want to use any hormone therapy, and removed the patch. Because my doctor stated that it was my option, she acquiesced.

Within an hour of my waking from the surgery, I sneezed and thought that I pulled a muscle. I was unable to move, and the pain was excruciating. I thought I had pulled a hernia in my side. I was wheeled into X-ray, but nothing obvious was found. After a couple of hours, the pain subsided and I was able to lay flat. Eventually I was allowed to go home, with no HRT patch and no pain, but also no more ability to have any more babies. I would not have any more babies of my body, but GOD blessed me with my own little miracle boy. Thank you. Life goes on.

As I thought back on the pain during my menstrual cycles, the amount of bleeding that occurred, the large amount of blood clotting, and the foul stench of decay associated with the clots that were being passed, I realized that I may have had any number of miscarriages prior to the birth of my little warrior. I had often wondered why my bleeding was so messy and heavy that I could only use Super Pads, while everyone else was complaining about finding the right size tampons. The foul odor of decay should have been a RED flag, because that is not normal. But I can admit today that I suffered from episodes of 'young and stupid' in my youth. It also didn't help that I was a child of an era in time where certain things were not discussed. And to tell someone that you are passing clotty, foul masses of tissue was embarrassing enough. If you have experienced any of this, GET IT CHECKED NOW.

Chapter 13   More Research/More Explanations

As I worked to keep my son healthy and away from allergic triggers, I realized that I had my own share of trigger demons to deal with. So, I started taking my own health issues much more seriously.

I was like everyone else. I expected to go to the doctor, and have them address every health problem that I had. I expected them to tell me that I had this problem or that, and it could be fixed with this medicine or that medicine. That is where we mess up. No one should seriously believe that every ailment you have, will be fixed with the stroke of a pen or the prescription of a drug. **It's Your Health – Own It**. After taking ownership of my baby's health issues, I finally started to take ownership of my own health problems. It was very enlightening.

The first thing I did was to go back to the food research that I'd so diligently performed for my son. I also decided to do another elimination diet. But, before I started the elimination diet, I wrote down most of the foods that I consumed with reckless abandonment. I have to admit I love to eat. And I had no problem with trying new things, so this newest elimination diet was like a drug withdrawal. I thought I was suffering from the DTs. DTs (Delirium Tremens) are the reaction to sudden drug or alcohol withdrawal, which can cause severe disturbance in the brain or to the nervous system. I truly did not have these problems, but I felt like I did. I like to eat. I made it through the Elimination Diet this time and learned some serious lessons. I want to share them with you.

Chapter 14 MSG (Monosodium Glutamate)

The first thing that I learned from my second elimination diet was that I should have paid better attention during my first elimination diet. It is truly amazing what the body can tell you about yourself, and how to take care of *you*. Listen to your body. There were so many hints back then. I could have saved myself a lot of headaches, literally.

As I mentioned, I could have saved myself a lot of headaches. I truly could have, because I suffered from migraines. My migraines were so severe, I thought that my head was going to explode (and not because it's so big). The pain was blinding and debilitating, and the medicine only made matters worse. I would have to lie down before the headache would go away. It would actually take me off of my feet.

I loved to eat Chinese food. Never had a problem with eating it, but that had a lot to do with where I got it from. Now that I wasn't moving around so much (I was in the military for nine years), I would eat at the same local restaurants. This helped me in isolating a new allergic trigger: MSG. MSG (Monosodium Glutamate) is the sodium salt of glutamic acid, one of the most abundant, naturally-occurring, non-essential amino acids. A lot of the Chinese restaurants that I had eaten at before did not use the flavor enhancer, however, others used it to enhance everything, and with reckless abandonment. We live in a world where salt is used to enhance the flavor of almost everything. I believed that the intensity of the sodium salt content in MSG contributed too much to the enhancement of my foods. The enhancement-MSG was a significant trigger in the migraines that I experienced. It was not the only trigger, I would eventually learn.

I mentioned earlier that, during my experience with Dairy, I suffered from headaches. Though not as severe as the migraines from MSG, the Dairy headaches were running a close second. Some of the other reactions to MSG and Dairy were similar to what I perceived to be 'stroke' symptoms. There would be sudden onset headaches, nausea, vomiting, and numbness. Other symptoms would have nothing to do with stroke. Those symptoms would be congestion, runny nose, difficulty swallowing and breathing, severe joint stiffness (arthritis- like), and chest pains. But the weirdest symptom associated with MSG was the feeling of a sub-dermal itch that you just can't scratch. Along with this itch, there's a feeling of something walking or crawling under your skin. It would feel as if there is an army of
nano-bugs or microscopic organisms crawling between the dermal layers of your skin. But it was a fungal attack of the body. The itchy feel would occur wherever the MSG touched me.

Say for instance, if I consumed a bag of potato chips that contained the ingredient MSG or Monosodium Glutamate, the hand in the bag would begin to itch, a very painful itch. More specifically, the very tips of my fingers would start an itch that is like a burning itch. It is almost hard to describe but trust me, if you have ever experienced this itch, you can relate to the misery it causes. Along with the itch, I would begin to develop a hacking cough and runny nose, then difficulty breathing. I would also develop an intense headache, and then my stomach would become upset. If I didn't make it to a bathroom immediately, bad things would happen. And the headaches would trigger a bout of nausea that would be so hard to contain that sleeping would be the only thing that helped.

I am so sensitive to MSG that I now am able to smell the ingredient long before I taste it. This is a good thing because some restaurants will use MSG in their foods, even when they say that they do not. If you are allergic to MSG or monosodium glutamate: be aware and be wary.

Chapter 15   Let's Sum it All Up

The information that I have provided is some of my family's allergy history. By no means am I downplaying the importance of doctors and their medical staff, scientists and their research, but, you must be involved in your health because it's yours, and you know or can learn the messages and warnings that your body sends out to you. And there are a lot of simple things that you can do to help yourself get through them.

First thing, if it doesn't feel right, don't do it. That goes with eating and drinking. If your body responds negatively, let it go. You don't need it. And if you have a serious response, don't ignore it. It only takes seconds/minutes to asphyxiate, so time is not on your side. If you feel an attack coming on, stay calm and attempt to relax. Excitability equals adrenaline rush, and adrenaline rush and respiratory stress, do not go together. CALM DOWN!!!

If you are seriously allergic, get that Epipen, but be mindful of the fact that the Epipen will not be cheap. My most recent purchase price for the Epipen was $473.99 prior to the insurance, and after insurance my out-of-pocket expense was $118.55 for a twin pack, and that twin pack was only good for one year. Make sure that you need it, and that you can afford it, because this will be one of your best lines of defense. Also, doctors will probably prescribe breathing treatments. These work well for acute and chronic respiratory problems, but I'm not sure of its effect on anaphylactic shock. Treatment for anaphylaxis should be immediate. As with any medical emergency, please STAY CALM, and in control.

Also, drink lots of water. I don't mean for you to drown yourself in it, but make sure you consume sufficient amounts of water per day. Water works wonders in diluting any mucus buildup in your system. Plain water, not designer water or water substitutes, just plain water. The water will help the mucus and congestion pass through your system, not allowing the mucus to stop and adhere itself to your bronchial tube lining. If the mucus is not moving, it starts to solidify and turns into snot or booggas or whatever crude word that you want to call it. You don't want it to sit in your system and block your passage. That's a disaster waiting to happen. Cough it up or blow it out, but get rid of the mucus, and water will definitely help slide it through. I have also found that with some children, patting their backs helps to loosen up to mucus blockage.

As a parent, whenever my son would show a reaction to an allergen, the first thing he would do was scratch, then his eyes would water; next he would have a very runny nose and his eyes would redden. Also, the lens' barrier of the eye would fill with liquid, and his eyes would drain. Next, he would begin to wheeze in his chest and start gasping for air. Scary, let me tell you. Trust me when I say that Actifed® and Sudafed® were life savers. I am not an abuser of medications, but when you see your baby in severe respiratory distress, your only concern is for their immediate relief, and you make it happen. Once the liquid took effect, he would be breathing normally, and I would always follow-up with a visit to the clinic to ensure that my son was okay or, depending on the severity of the incident, take him to the emergency room.

I was a little apprehensive about pediatric clinics because at the time, if you brought your child in with respiratory problems, you would be signed in and would wait for long periods of time. This happened quite often for my son until one particular incident that set his pediatrician off.

My son had a reaction and I rushed him to the clinic. He had an appointment with his pediatrician for later that day, but we could not wait. I checked him in for respiratory distress and waited, and waited, and waited to see a doctor. After over an hour of waiting, I decided to take him to the emergency room but needed to cancel his pediatric appointment, because I could not stay for it. It just so happens that his pediatrician's office was in the same building and on the same floor as the clinic, and his pediatrician was in the lobby at the time we arrived to cancel. She immediately assessed the situation, administered treatment and then asked how he got to be in this state.

I told her that he had a reaction at home and I took him to the clinic in this building, because it had not gotten too severe yet. When I informed the receptionist that he was having breathing difficulties, she told us to have a seat, and we would be called. That was almost two hours ago, and he became progressively worse, so I decided to take him to the emergency. Well, when his doctor checked him out she informed me that, from now on, when he arrives at that clinic for respiratory distress, he will be taken back immediately. My son would not have to wait another second longer. And she was right, because after she politely corrected the clinic personnel on issues pertaining to respiratory distress and children, he never waited for treatment. And when I say immediate response, I mean immediate. For your child's sake, get their doctors involved, because a doctor can move medical mountains that you may perceive as too difficult for you to climb.

I learned a lot about symptoms and signs, but one of the most distinct indicators of allergic response was for Peanut butter. My son was so sensitive to Peanut butter that, whenever the seal of a Peanut butter container was opened, the essence was enough to trigger all of the reactions mentioned above. His reaction was so immediate and severe that, whenever Peanut butter sandwiches were prepared for the other children at his daycare, he would be removed from the area to eat his meals with the center's director. The first time his daycare providers experienced his reaction, most of them were in tears. To see a small child appear as if someone physically brutalized them would bring a grown person to their knees, and my son was no exception. But one of the things that I did was to ensure them that they did no wrong by him. I also reminded them that if he can breathe without difficulty, just call me, but if his breathing is distressed, call 911 and then call me.

I remember one time when we were on an airplane and the flight attendant was passing out the standard '3-peanuts-in-bag' snack to all of the passengers. I politely thanked her and handed our bags back, informing her that my son was allergic to peanuts. She immediately went back through the entire airplane, taking the snack bags back from the passengers and replacing them with pretzels. The attendant was very mindful of the fact that anything in the aircraft's air will recirculate, including peanut dust/essence, and if there is one person allergic to nuts, there is the potential for an in-flight medical alert. That flight attendant was trained well.

There was also an episode where one of my son's cousins gave him a Peanut M&M. At the time, my son was about 3-years old and one of his favorite snacks was plain M&Ms. He begged his cousin for one of hers, not knowing that M&Ms could contain peanuts, and she was not aware of his nut allergies. By the time he got to me, he could barely breathe. I checked his breath and it reeked of Peanuts. My immediate response was to give him a dose of Actifed®. I did not know how severe his reaction was until the

Actifed® worked, he threw up his stomach content, and normal breathing returned.

Today, my son is still sensitive to nuts (all nuts) but not as sensitive as he was as a small child. Before, you could not eat any nuts within his airspace, now it doesn't bother him. But, if nuts have become rancid and my son touches them, he will have an allergic reaction. When nuts turn Rancid, the fats or oils from the nuts decompose, emitting a strong odor and rendering them not suitable for consumption. Now in 2015, the oil or fat of the nut is my son's allergic trigger, so that means no foods prepared in Peanut Oil. He can smell it but cannot touch it, which is an enormous improvement.

I mentioned earlier in the book that my son is allergic to Soy. Well, he got it from his mom. I know that whenever I changed my son's diaper, during the period that he consumed Soy Baby formula, the smell would trigger a 'gag' response from me, but I thought that it was just because of the smell. His stool would have a very sweet smell that was nauseating. But I found out later in life just how allergic I was to Soy. I joined LA Weight Loss because I wanted to lose a few pounds. Their advertisement got me in the door, but as soon as I signed up I was told that, in order to obtain the weight loss that I was expecting, I had to use their foods and supplements. When I started the program, my blood pressure was normal and my weight was okay, but I still needed to lose the extra pounds. Well, by the end of the month, my blood pressure was so high that I wound up on blood pressure medication, I was gaining weight, and I was bloated and congested. Finally, I read the labels on the items that I was required to eat, and found that everything contained Soy.

After quitting the program, a couple weeks went by and the bloating subsided, I dropped a couple of pounds, but my pressure was too far gone for me to get off of the medication. I've been on blood pressure medicine, ever since.

As far as my Dairy allergy is concerned, I was not always allergic to dairy. I remember a hundred years ago when I was a little child, we lived in the projects. My dad had a friend who would give him bottles of raw milk that was truly some good stuff. I remember drinking only raw milk until around the age of ten, when my parents could afford to go to the local A&P and purchase pasteurized milk. Because the local grocery store was just across the street from the projects, we had milk available whenever we needed it. Not too long after that I began to suffer from respiratory problems, and every type of ailment became much harder to deal with. I remember suffering from a very severe case of Chicken Pox, that caused my parents to keep me confined inside for an entire week. And when I was able to leave the house, it was only to sit outside in the sun, wrapped in blankets, like a cocoon. I was always congested, coughing up heavy mucus. And then the dreaded menstrual cycle began and it all went downhill with a swiftness that was unimaginable. Now that I look back on that time, I think I began to suffer from Dairy allergies back then, but I could not understand what was different between the two sources of milk. The only thing that I can think of is the containerization of the dairy, for transport. You cannot move that much product without missing something and I think that the something that was missing was the total sterilization of the containers used to move the milk. Although pasteurization is performed on the milk that we consume, how are the containers treated that move the milk from the cows to the stores? Pasteurization heats the product to a high enough temperature to kill off microorganisms, but is the sterilization process for any and all of the containers at one hundred percent? If this step is not taken seriously, it will only take the release of one group of spores to cause the problems that I have with milk. And once the spore is in the body, it can lay dormant until a new trigger occurs. FOOD FOR THOUGHT

I always like to say that the average teenager thinks that they are bulletproof: can do anything, eat anything, say anything, and get away with everything. But think about it. We were all in that position at some time in our life, and some adults still believe that they are. Nothing wrong with that, but if you're going to be like that about the things you do, be realistic about it. You are not a teenager anymore, and even if you did not have allergies or did not recognize them as allergic reactions in your youth, they may very well be allergies that you are dealing with now. And don't believe that since you use to be able to eat this, or drink that, you can still do it without being ill. A lot of the illnesses that we may contribute to one thing, could very well be your body's response to histamine triggers, defining a problem that you need to be aware of. Allergic reactions can be as simple as a urinary tract infection, yeast infection, or runny nose, to chest congestion and wheezing, or as severe as anaphylactic shock and death. Know your body. And if you are experiencing a severe allergic reaction, seek immediate medical attention. Stay calm and drink that water!!!

Chapter 16 Bottom Line

The bottom line is simple: you are the custodian of your body. And for some of us, we are the custodians of others charged to our care. We have also been extremely blessed with medical support and scientific advantages that are well beyond the wildest of imaginations. But your body and your health are just that: YOURS. Acknowledge your health and take ownership. Take the time to look at yourself and your symptoms. Have that detailed discussion with your doctors, but know that you are the first line of defense with your health, so OWN that responsibility and never take it for granted. Don't leave your health in the hands of prescriptions and assumptions.

Remedies along the Way

First and foremost – **WATER. Drinking good, old fashion H$_2$O has major benefits for the body. Water not only helps to flush out and move the bad mucus and impurities through your system, but it helps the bodies' natural filters to flush out toxins that are always associated with allergies. If you ever have a severe allergic reaction, but you are not near medical help, stay calm and slowly drink some water until help arrives or you reach medical help. The water will help to lubricate the throat area, liquefying the mucus buildup. And staying calm helps to keep the adrenaline rush down.

Coconut Oil

I have some of the worse skin, or at least I use to have. My face is very oily but the rest of my body is extremely dry, and the older I get, the worse it has gotten. But in the last few years, I have found a new best product for both my oily face and my extreme dry skin: Coconut Oil, great for the entire body, from head to toe, and all areas in between. In the warmer months, I use coconut oil as a body moisturizer. One of the things that amazed me was how effective coconut oil is on oily skin. I have very oily facial skin, and was very reluctant to put anything on it for fear of aggravating the skin and producing more oil. But as I have aged, so has my skin and mature skin needs protection.

My skin is still oily but at night, I wear a layer of coconut oil on my face and neckline, and have found that not only has my skin improved, but the coconut oil keeps the bed linen from 'wicking out' the natural oils from my skin. Coconut oil has helped to balance out my skin, from head to toe. That may have a lot to do with coconut oil's natural antifungal and antibacterial effect. Can't go wrong there. And a big 54 ounce jar will run you less than $16.00, and lasts for a very long time. The one I use is Carrington Farms Coconut Oil, sold at Costco. When your money is low, you can't beat Coconut Oil for its value and its uses. It can safely be used on a baby's delicate skin and hair, as well. Another good coconut oil product is called MONOi Tiki Tahiti®. This product is made in Tahiti, but I found it at VITACOST website. VITACOST is a great website for a lot of the products mentioned in this book, and the prices are extremely reasonable. But, back to the MONOi Tiki Tahiti® oil. This oil is so effective that it can be used on some of the driest of skin and hair, with great results, and it only has four ingredients- coconut oil Tiare (Gardenia tahitensis), fragrance, and Vitamin E. It comes in a 4 fluid ounce (120 ml) container and cost a couple of dollars, but if you can afford it, it's worth it. If you can't afford it, plain, old coconut oil works great and is much cheaper.

One more thing about Coconut Oils, there are a lot of

products that are not what they seem are advertise. Be careful. You may think that you have Coconut Oil, but you have an oil blend, instead. One sure fire way of knowing if you got the right one is, if someone comes to you hungry, and the first thing they mention is that they wants some fried chicken, then chances are you are wearing a coconut oil blend. But if a hungry person mentions that they could eat an **ALMOND JOY®** or a **MOUND®** bar when they approach you, then you got the right oil.

Shea Butter

But when the winter comes and the air is dryer, my body craves a little more protection. I have found one of the best protections for both hair and skin in a jar of Shea Butter. Whoever brought Shea Butter to the mass population: THANK YOU!!! I use Shea Butter when the humidity is at its lowest, and the air is at its driest and coldest. It takes a little work to get it warmed up for use, but once you've rubbed it together and are ready to use it, you will not regret it. It works on Eczema, those little bumps on the arms, rough knees and elbows, and even in your hair. A jar can last you through the roughest of winters, making your skin feel new-born, baby-soft. But it's just as effective when the months warm up. And the protection that Shea Butter provides is priceless. Don't get frustrated; just keep rubbing it together.

Tamanu

When my son was a baby and for many years afterwards, I would use this one product for his Eczema and dry skin: Tamanu. My son's Eczema was so severe, his skin felt like textured paint on the wall. That's the best way to describe it. I felt like I needed to chisel a layer of skin off to reach the smoother layer. After all of the research that I completed, I still needed to do more, and eventually found this one product call Tamanu. The one that I used came in a cream form called True Tamanu®. I'm not sure if it's still for sale, but it was the only thing that worked to smooth away the textured feeling, while moisturizing my son's skin. This is Mother Nature at her best.

Underarm Odor

Another favorite item did not show up until my son was much older. As any person transitions from toddler to puberty, things change. But one of the most distinct changes happen under the arm pits. We all know it for the odor that it is, and no one is immune to it. And since my son was so allergic but still experienced the change, I wanted something that was very effective yet bearable, and we found it: THAI® Crystal Deodorant Mist. This is one of the most effective deodorants I have ever used. It contains purified water and mineral salts; that's it, yet it controls underarm odor with just a few sprays. I needed to find something that was not heavy or pore- clogging, and this is it. A friend mentioned how effective it was for his family and I decided to try it. It works great, and one bottle lasts a long time. THAI® Crystal Deodorant comes in a solid, as well, but the solid is an actual solid piece of mineral salt and nothing else. Both solid and mist are extremely effective, and with only two ingredients in the mist and one in the solid, you know exactly what you are using.

Fever Blisters and Cold Sores

Fever blisters (or cold sores) are a common occurrence for many people, but they are an ugly sight to see, for anyone. We do what we can to cover them up and try everything possible to eliminate them. But, because of what they are, keeping control of the flare-ups takes a bit of work. I experience them like lots of other people, but the way I handle them may be different from others but most effective for me. When I feel that unmistakable tingle around my lips and under the skin, I hold an alcohol swab over the area for a minute, or until the sting goes away. Then I apply a layer of CARMEX® original lip balm. I do this, two or three times per day and usually the flare-up, or potential threat of a flare-up, is gone by the next day. It really works and cost pennies to do. I suspect that if you're brave enough, it may work on genital flare-ups as well, but I am not suggesting using it because the alcohol effect is unforgiving and the CARMEX® will give you an enticing little tingle.

Hemorrhoids

Hemorrhoids are a fact of life for a lot of people. They are that dirty little secret we try to avoid discussing but they occur, especially during pregnancy. The best way to handle external hemorrhoids is to keep the area clean and free of moisture. The moisture in the anal area is a breeding ground for bacteria and, if you do not keep this area clean, it will aggravate the skin and breed all kinds of *things*. When you bathe, check your body folds to see if the body odor has been eliminated. Sometimes we think that because we have showered or bathe well, that we have taken care of everything, yet, in the folds of our bodies, bacteria may linger. Smell yourself and if you smell clean, you have accomplished your mission. But if you smell yourself and you still smell a hint of B.O., clean it again. Once you feel confident that the odor has been eliminated, you're done. And if you are worried about not having enough moisture in those special areas, apply a thin layer of coconut oil. Coconut oil will provide that barrier, and it's a natural anti- bacterial and anti-fungal, which will help to keep the bacteria down and the body odor 'at bay'.

The stress and strain that may trigger internal hemorrhoids can be minimize by increasing your intact of fiber (and not the sugared kind), just plain, old fiber. Fiber from your foods is the best source, but there are other forms of fiber that may help. But all fibers work best when accompanied by a large glass of water. Always get your water 'fix'. You don't have to swim in it but get a good dosing of water, daily. It is your best all- around dietary benefit. My preference in fiber supplement is one that has nothing but the fiber in it. You don't need anything that makes it taste good or easier to swallow. If you mix it well, the swallowing is not noticeable, and if you don't like the bland flavor, mix it with a juice. Remember that you are not drinking it because it tastes like your favorite beverage; you're drinking it to increase your fiber intake, and assist your digestion with processing your food through your system.

On the subject of adding fiber to your diet, psyllium husk and glucomannan are soluble fibers that absorb moisture and take on a gel-like state. In this state, the fibers help with pushing the trash out of your body, and by binding to garbage that may get stuck in your digestive system's hidden side pockets, and dragging it out with the rest of the trash. Trust me, when you take in the right fiber, you will see a big and positive difference in your fecal (stool) production

---

Shingles

During a period in my life when I wasn't feeling my best, and my immunities were extremely low, I caught some crazy virus. The virus weakened my immunities even more and I wound up with Bronchitis. After the Bronchitis was over, I got Shingles. When it rains, it pours. And let me tell you that once you get Shingles, you don't want to ever get it again. Shingles started off as a severe pain across my back that started moving to the front of my body. At the same time a rash appeared over my left breast. I really didn't think much about the pain and the rash working together until the rash began to get worse, and the pain increased. I went to see a Dermatologist who prescribed Desoximetasone® Gel USP, 0.05%. I was told to use this three times per day. Immediately upon placing the gel on the rash, the pain was excruciating. Every time that I applied the Gel, the rash was screaming with pain. I did this for two weeks but the rash got worse and the pain was relentless. Finally, I went to my General Practitioner and she immediately informed me that I had Shingles. Can it get any worse? I was given an antibiotic and was told that I should continue to use the Gel until the rash heals. The rash did not heal, and for weeks I suffered. Finally, I made my own cream. Not only did the cream calm the nerve endings immediately, but the rash began to go away. It may or may not work for you, but it was and continues to be, one of the best concoctions that I have ever used. As a matter of fact, if I have the feeling that comes with the onset of Shingles, I immediately apply the cream and the sensation goes away. The cream I used is a combination of Coconut Oil, Shea Butter, Avocado Oil, and Neem Oil. Depending on the size of the container that you use, mix 2 parts Shea Butter; 1½ parts Coconut Oil; 2 Tablespoons Avocado Oil; 1 Tablespoons Neem Oil. In order to mix the items, they will need to be in liquid form, and how I accomplish this is to microwave slowly or melt them on top of the stove. DO NOT BOIL OR OVERHEAT, JUST MELT and remove from heat. Once the combination has turned to liquid, just stir it up until you feel that it is mixed well. Cover the product and place in the freezer. Once it freezes solid, remove from freezer and use. When it thaws, the texture should remain consistent with creams, and it will be very easy to use. The combination works so well, I use it for any skin flare-ups, as well as when my skin feels a bit drier.

Stye

Before I reached adulthood, I had multiple episodes with Stye. Stye is a painful inflammation on or around the eyelid. I was prescribed eyeglasses to eliminate the problem, which only made it worse. Eventually, I realized that the best way to handle the abscess was with a warm washcloth over the inflamed area and a mild pain reliever (aspirin, Naprosyn, Tylenol, etc.). The cloth removed the pressure and sting from the eye area, and the pain reliever helped to remove the internal pain.

Conjunctivitis or Pinkeye

My son experienced a couple of episodes of Conjunctivitis before I realized that the prescribed treatment wasn't working for him. Conjunctivitis (or Pinkeye) is the inflammation of the conjunctiva. Conjunctiva is the thin, clear layer of the white area of the eye. For Conjunctivitis, there was a LOT of crusty mucus buildup and the work was a little more intense. The biggest thing is to remove the mucus from the infected area. You can do this by applying a very warm and damp washcloth/rag over the area. The warmth and the moistures help to loosen the dried, 'caking effect' of the mucus over the eyes. Lightly remove the crusty mucus, washing your hands throughout the process. Clean the area around the eyes and make sure that you and your children clean your hands at all times. Cleanliness is the best and first line of defense. Keep the eye area clean with a warm, damp, clean washcloth. Always use a clean, unused washcloth, and always wash your hand and your child's hands, as well. And keep the face clean.

Natural Pesticide

Have you ever wondered about the contents of the insect sprays that you use around your family? I did, but was limited in what was available until one day, over fifteen years ago. We are always telling our children to not take food into their rooms because it may attract bugs. Well, it's kind of hard to keep a toddler focused on not taking stuff into their rooms. They're so busy playing, they are not thinking about too much else. One day, when my son was taking a nap, I noticed a line on the wall in his room. I thought that he'd drawn the line, but it was too high on the wall for his height. Upon closer inspection, I realized that it was not a line, but a trail of ants marching from the window to a cup of juice on his night stand.

Since my son was napping on my bed, I took the opportunity to spray insecticide on the ant trail in his room. At least I thought that I was going to use insecticide, but I didn't have any on hand. I did have a can of BLUE MAGIC Pure® Citrus Oil Air Freshener, and so I sprayed that and walked away. Well, when I returned to the room not two minutes later, the trail was dead. What the heck –it was a spray; it was in a can; who knew?? From that day forward, whenever there was a need for insecticide treatments, I would spray BLUE MAGIC Pure® Citrus Oil Air Freshener. It works on spiders, flies, ants (of course), roaches, mosquitos, and whatever creepy bug you may run across. I was even tempted to use it on snakes, but I dared not get close enough to try. So, if your child is not allergic to citrus, this is a great insecticide to use around children, pets, and plants, with no side effects. It's not as potent as insecticides, but that's okay, because I'm not trying to knock myself out when I knock the bugs out. If I need something stronger, then I will use something stronger. But, try the Orange spray out and see for yourself.

Hot Flashes

I mentioned in an earlier chapter that I had had a Hysterectomy. One of the things about a Hysterectomy is that, eventually, you will be forced through a pre-mature menopause. Either pre-maturely or during the regular course of a woman's life cycle if we live long enough, we all will experience some level of menopausal symptoms. And I was no different. The one difference is that my cycle only lasted about two weeks and then, the obvious symptoms were gone. I experienced the hot flashes, night sweats, irritability, and many other typical symptoms of menopause but, because of my observations of my reactions to food, I was able to understand some of the triggers for some of my menopausal reactions. One of the triggers was the over-consumption of carbohydrates and sugars. Certain cravings tend to increase and I was acting upon them, and my body was telling me NO. When I consumed products with sugar or empty carbs, I would suffer from severe hot flashes and night sweats or chills. I thought that I was going crazy. But once I cut back on those items - no more flashes, night sweat, or chills. Even if I prepared the item myself from scratch, and it contained too much sugar or flour, I would react. Also, too much pasta was no good for me, and sodas were taboo. Anything that contained a lot of carbs would put me into menopausal distress, and they also contributed to my belly fat and weight gain. And trust me when I say that it is miserable when you are now overweight when you were once a small size and also waking up in the middle of the night drenched in sweat; or stopping in the middle of whatever you are doing to strip your clothes off (and it could get you arrested in some places).

CHEW your Food

As we get older, it seems like our bodies start to fall apart. If it's not one ailment, it's something else, so when I started having severe pains in my upper stomach area, I went straight to the internet. I checked all my symptoms and, wouldn't you know it, I was experiencing classic symptoms of EVERYTHING. With too many ailments for the stomach problem, I turned to a Gastroenterologist. After months of testing and pouring what little money I had into the bottomless pit of medical fees, the diagnoses was simple – we can't find anything wrong. Now mind you, I was suffering some serious pains, to the point that I could not sleep. The pain was there when I ate or when I slept; when I walked or when I exercised; when I worked or did absolutely nothing; I was in pain. Yet the doctor could find no problem and all of my digestive tract area was operating, normally. Okay, now what??? So I spent some time thinking and reading, and thinking and reading. Finally, after all of that brain work, I experienced an "ah hah" moment. It was that moment when I realized that I can truly be an idiot. What is it that your mom tells you as a little kid; "CHEW ALL OF YOUR FOOD BEFORE YOUR SWALLOW".

I have stated this to my son often, but wasn't practicing what I preached. For whatever reason (and it was not a good one), I was not chewing my food thoroughly. The digestive process requires that we provide assistance at the mouth entry. It's not that much work; just chew everything that is chewable, until it becomes more liquid than solid. And for that little bit of effort, your digestive tract will work much more efficiently. Chewing will break down the rest of your food for your body's benefit. And in return, you get all the nutrients you need to sustain a healthy life. Once that little tidbit registered in my tiny, little mind, the rest was gravy, literally. NO MORE PAIN. If the pain reoccurs, I think back to what I just consumed, lubricate my system with water, and relax. Remember, the digestive system contains some narrow paths that can clog. Just like the plumbing system in your home. Or, just think about the straw that you may use. The narrow passageway of a straw will accommodate apple juice easily, but not the whole apple or apple slices. CHEW YOUR FOOD thoroughly.

Vertigo

I suffer from Vertigo. My episodes can be pretty severe. There is nothing like going on a magical ride that you didn't sign up for.

When I was little, I was the child who watched everybody else on the Fair rides. All it takes is one ride full of vomit to let you know that you can't do that anymore. But as I got older, I could go on some rides as long as I didn't eat before the journey. Yet, it only takes one mishap to change everything. And my one mishap occurred when I was in the military. As I entered a military cargo plane, I bumped my head on a metal rod that was protruding over the entryway. Man that hurt but, being in the military, you shake it off and keep it moving. A few months later, my husband and I are staying in a hotel with a waterbed. I'm excited thinking that this will be the best sleep ever. Let me tell you, I am so glad that I never purchased a waterbed for my home because, after spending a night in one, it turned my world upside down, literally. I had to roll out of bed, to get out of it. As soon as I stood up, I tilted over. Everything was moving and so was I, because I could not walk and had to be taken to the emergency room. The on-duty doctor could find nothing wrong but told me that there was something going on and I would need to see my primary doctor. I did and received a diagnosis of Vertigo. I was given a prescription of Meclizine hydrochloride. I'm not sure which was worse, the ailment or the cure, because the medicine had me just as loopy as the Vertigo. As time passed, I experienced intermittent episodes of Vertigo. There was never a 'rhyme or reason' behind any one episode and the triggers were always different. It could a virus or bad food; sitting up too quickly or lying flat; talking or walking; driving or riding; you name it and it could trigger it. I would take the Meclizine and it would work, but my quality of life was 'suspect'. I was less functional whenever I would take the medicine. My sister and I went on a cruise vacation one year. While on the cruise ship, we ran into some rough waters. The ride didn't bother my sister but I experienced a severe bout of Vertigo. The Meclizine worked, but I was too drugged to enjoy the rest of the trip. This did not make for a fun journey. Eventually, I wanted to go on another cruise vacation but was terrified of my Vertigo reactions. I went to the drugstores and grocery stores looking for a motion sickness product that contained the smallest amount of Meclizine or whatever motion sickness medicine available. Low and behold, I came across a couple of armband motion sickness products. But one stood out. This particular armband product contained NO DRUGS whatsoever. Now really, I consider myself to be fairly intelligent and am I supposed to believe that a band with NO DRUGS in it will stop my motion sickness? Somebody is trying to pull a fast one on the public by peddling the newest 'snake oil' product. Okay, so why not give it a try - once. But I had a backup – The trusty, reliable, headache- inducing Meclizine. So I went on another cruise. Let me tell you, those armbands were unbelievable. The boat was rocking and so was I. I set on my balcony during an approaching storm and enjoyed the view (until I got drenched). My cabin was on the 9th deck and the boat was rocking and the water was splashing all the way up past my balcony. That was okay with me because that was the best I had felt in a long time. I still have the bands and have not had to use them since. But if I have another bout of Vertigo, anywhere, I will put them on and 'rock the boat' again. The bands that I am referring to are by Sea-Band®. The price varies but I purchased mine for $8.99. At first, I was reluctant to pay this price. But now, it was one of the best investments that I could have made. And the beauty of the bands is that they are washable – up to five times. Can you beat that? NOPE.

Morning Nasal congestion

One of the simplest things that a person can do to relieve nasal passage congestion is to give your nose a good blow. I don't mean to blow your brains out through your nose, but to give your nostrils a good, cleansing blow, especially in the morning when you get up. When I get up in the morning, there are times that I may be congested. After a night's sleep, mucus will sometimes settle in my sinus passage. When I get out of bed and begin to get my day going, the mucus shifts and starts to become released from its slumber; my head becomes a little congested and my sinuses start to drain. So what I do is I place a slight pressure on one side of my nose and massage; then I will do the same to the other side; and then I will hold both sides(with a tissue) and give myself a good, hearty blow. I may have to do this a couple of times, but eventually that mucus will come out. And if there is any clogging going on, this will come out also. Then I move on with my day. Now I can breath and my sinus passage is clear for the rest of the day.

There are lots of great products out there that have very few ingredients but work just as well as any other product (if not better); you just have to take a little time to check them out.
GOOD LUCK!!!

[[We live in a world of fear. Fear of loving, fear of laughing, fear of enjoying the fruits of our labor. Don't live in fear of people with health issues that you do not understand. Ask the questions; have the conversations; learn and understand.

If you see someone with a fever blister or Pinkeye, don't assume that they are going to transmit it to you. Truth be told, if you were one of those 'snotty-nosed brats like I was, you probably got the spore living dormant in your system. And having allergies make them worse. Everything can be handled where it does not transmit to others, and there are ways of keeping them under control without breaking the bank or taking medications that have severe side effects. Investigate and shop around. You would be amazed at how easy and readily available the knowledge is to you.]]

I can hear you saying to yourself that this person has experienced more health problems than a medical book contains. It may sound that way, but I believe that I am in tune to what happens with my body. It's not hurting me to share my experiences with you and who knows who I may help, so why not put the information in a book for others to read.

Out of everything that I have suggested, the best remedy and suggestion that I could give a parent of a child with food allergies, is to be willing to cook your own meals. Even if you cannot cook, it will not take much to learn. You don't have to be the world's next top master chef, or even pay a school to provide you with lessons so that you gain a doctorate degree in culinary arts; just experiment with what you have available to you. All you need to do is be able to prepare your meals with basic ingredients. Simple Fare - nothing fancy. You would be amazed at your own abilities. You can control the price of each meal and stay within your budget, while preparing a mouth-watering meal made with your own little hands that your whole family will love. Stay away from processed foods because you don't know what every package contains. But, if you prepare your meals from scratch, you will at least have a basic knowledge of the ingredients in the meals you and your family will be eating. BON APPETIT!!!

IMPORTANT
(Heart Health)

Before I close out this book, I wanted to speak on one other issue. As a baby, my son experienced a severe case of Chicken Pox. During this time, he maintained a fever that was constantly over 102.7°. He was given Amoxicillin, but the fever would not break. After five straight days of this, I demanded that he be given a different antibiotic that I knew would work for him. Two hours after receiving his first dose of the other antibiotic his fever broke, and a couple days later, he was back to his old self – or was he?

As time passed, I became concerned that my son would suffer from heart problems and brain abnormalities due to the prolonged high fever. My concern was not so much for his brain activities, because my son was and still is a bright person, but I worried about his heart. Yet, I did nothing. Finally, I decided that he needed to be tested and explained to his doctor my reasons why. I told them of his long period with a high fever, and his father's heart health issues. My son was given a three-dimensional heart health scan, at a 'satellite site' for Children's Health Care of Atlanta. This was amazing to watch, but the results proved that, unless he had some other difficulty that may transpire later in life, my son's heart was very healthy. What a relief that was – until I got the bill. Even with health care insurance, my out-of-pocket expense was $525 for the scan. This is not something that everyone can afford to pay out-of-pocket. It took me a couple of notices, and when I got the threatening notice stating that it was my FINAL NOTICE, I was glad of it. Okay, so I eventually paid it. But the satisfaction gained from knowing that my child's heart was healthy was worth it.

The reason why I bring this up is because many children have died from heart issues that no one knew existed. Knowing is half of the battle, and if a parent knows that their child may have heart health issues, they have the ability to do something about it. But when a parent watches their child drop dead before their eyes, from a heart ailment that could have been prevented, that is devastating. A baseline heart scan should be a part of all Well-baby/Child care health assessments. If the initial scan is a part of Well-Child physicals, the cost to the parent would be covered by the insurance, and the knowledge would be in the parents' hands, to address the best that they can. Know your child's health risks early, because it could be a matter of a child's life or death. I just wanted this stated.

"As a doctor, I generalize, but as a parent, you specialize in your son's health." That statement from my baby's pediatrician still stays with me today, and it's because of that statement that I do not leave my health, or the health of my family in anyone else's hands but ours.

The Four Most Powerful Food Allergens
Experienced by my family
And their side effects

Dairy

Joint aches; congestion/respiratory distress; body aches; stomach cramping; blotting; headaches/migraines; night sweats; stiff neck; lockjaw; increased blood pressure; potential anaphylactic reaction; wheezing; conjunctivitis and/or Stye; itch, scaly skin; urinary tract infection; yeast infection; weight gain

Soy

Migraines; respiratory distress; runny nose; extreme increases blood pressure; congestion; explosive diarrhea; stomach problems; anaphylaxis; fever; weight gain; bloat

Peanut/Nut Products

Severe respiratory distress; severe anaphylaxis; runny nose/sinus drip; wheezing; chest congestion; watery eyes; conjunctivitis; fever; hives; rash; itchy, scaly skin

MSG (monosodium Glutamate)	Severe migraines; increased blood pressure; explosive, uncontrollable diarrhea; wheezing; chest congestion; respiratory distress; bloat and weight gain

IT'S YOUR HEALTH
Take Charge and Own It

FYI Some of the least observed but more common allergic responses could very well be arthritis and/or joint inflammation, gout, urinary tract infection, yeast infections, dandruff, nausea, and chronic pain. If you experience sudden onset of any of the above mentioned responses, check your diet. You could have an allergy that you may not have had before.

Our bodies change and we need to be able to accept the change. What we consumed before may not be consumable now; what medications we have taken in the past, our bodies may now be rejecting. Don't look at it as a 'death sentence' just because you can't eat what you use to be able to. Accept the change and move on with it. Consider it as a small negative in a world of so many positives. There are bigger issues in life that you're going to have to deal with, besides your favorite meal hating your guts.

*DEPENDING ON THE SEVERITY OF ANY ALLERGIC REACTIONS, ANAPHYLACTIC SHOCK AND EVEN DEATH MAY OCCUR.

Notes

_____

_____

_____

ABOUT THE AUTHOR

Born in Wilmington, North Carolina, Vandester Jenkins has spent her adult
life working in locations outside of North Carolina. She has spent over
nine years with the US Air Force as an Airman Integrated Avionics
Computer Specialist, and over twenty years as a Telecommunications and
Communications Maintenance Specialist, and Maintenance Supervisor. In
her travels, her careers have allowed her to not only meet a lot of special
and intriguing people, but gain a wealth of life experiences on how to deal
with them. She identifies that her most important experience has been that
of a mom, which has taught her that her experience in dealing with people
in general, are the foundation for the **P**atience, **P**ersistence, and
Perseverance she attempts to demonstrate at all times, when deal effectively
with her own son and his allergies and illnesses.